I0429263

Building Your Zero Fat Lean Muscle Belly

Simple Abs Muscle Workout Training Exercise Routines for Women

by Daniel Agbetorwoka

Published in United Kingdom by:

TKSD Publishing Ltd
Innovation Centre Medway
Maidstone Road, Chatham
Kent ME5 9FD

ISBN-**13: 978-1523435081**

ISBN-**10:1523435089**

Table of Contents

Introduction

Discover Why You Cannot Lose Weight Just By Exercising Alone

If you want to get rid of your fat belly or feel more energetic and take control of your fitness level but believed it was all impossible…then you need to read this book to the end.

When you do, you'll soon find out how it is all possible. You can get rid of your fat belly, feel more energetic and even enhance your fitness level. It's all possible. That's why this is the most valuable book you'll ever read!

Here's why … you now have a chance knowing that those feelings and worries will be short-lived. I can assure you that there is a simpler way to get rid of your stomach and body fat.

You can only discover that simpler way by getting the full copy of this book. Once you read it, you'll know the training and the routines you can do to burn your body fat and enhance your fitness level within 28 days.

The exercises and the workout routines you are going to read about in a moment are designed and tested to help anyone who wants to reduce their body weight and stomach fat. What is most important is to do so without having to resort to any restrictive special diets or training regimes.

With a bit of motivation on your part, you will learn to do simple muscle training routines to help you achieve your goal of having the perfect body and belly that you desired.

So what exactly are you going to learn and gain by reading this book?

First this book is different from others that you have read in the past. And this is why. As you read this book, you will also be able to access links to free **video scripts** that show you the exercises you read about. Not only that you will be able to read and learn these exercises and routines, you will also be able to watch them done live in the videos.

I am not paid for having links to these videos in the book. I put these links to the videos purposely for you to enhance your reading experience and to help you achieve your goals. Please watch these videos.

By reading the book and watching the videos, I believe you will gain all the benefits which you deserve in return for your decision to buy this book. At the end of the book, you will also find on the three bonus pages - **three free cheat sheets** that I have specially written for you, to accelerate your efforts to achieve the perfect body and zero fat belly that you desired.

With that said, what exactly are you going to learn or gain when you get a copy of this book? Here some of what you'll learn and the benefits.

1. **Discover Why Most People Cannot Lose Weight Even If They Exercise Regularly**.

2. How Carrying Excess Weight Around Certain Area of Your Body Can Result To A Serious Medical Condition

3. **How An Essential Nutrient In Your Diet Can Burn Your Belly Fat**

4. If You Read Nothing Else … Read Chapter Two!

5. **Do You Know The Two Types of Foods You Must Eliminate From Your Diet At All Cost If You Want A Lean Hard Zero Fat Belly?**

6. Do You Know Which Drinks You Must Avoid, If You are Really Serious about Building a Flat Slim Belly?

7. **A Little Secret to Curb Your Appetite So That You Eat Less Without Having to Go on a Diet**

8. The Two Must-Do Muscle Building Exercises.

9. **How A Simple Leg Exercise Can Flatten Your Abdominal Muscles**

10. The Simple Way to Fast-Track Losing Your Belly Fat If You're Overweight

11. **Five Effective Cardio Exercises and the Best Times to Do Them During The Day.**

12. The Simple, Step by step Training Routines that will make your Belly Muscles Hard-Rock Solid.

13. **The Secret of This 75 Years Old Dance Routines … How You Can Copy The Routines And Flatten Your Belly within Days**

14. And many more

Chapter 1:

Do You Want Zero Fat Belly? You Need Only One Thing to Succeed – It's Neither Exercise or a Diet

Do you know anyone who has a flat slim belly? Or have you seen a picture of someone who has what is popularly called a perfect six pack abs (men) and in women known as a zero fat belly, which you envy?

Is this something that interests you and you'll want one? As this book is written specifically for women, though men can also benefit if they choose to read it, this is what exactly a six back abs is and what it means…

A perfect six pack abs is when your abdominal muscles are so defined that they can be clearly seen. If you have a six pack stomach your muscles are well defined and you will be able to pick them out. There are six of them - three on each side of your abdomen and each one should look pronounced. Men sought to have the perfect six pack abs than women.

This is not to say that women should not try to achieve perfect six pack abs or zero fat belly. Women tend to worry more about having a flat slim stomach than men. But generally women tend to have soft looking bodies, which are not bulky with a muscular look like men.

You can also achieve perfect looking bulky or flat abdominal muscles if you follow the methods or the exercise routines I am going to show you in this guide.

But here is an advice. You shouldn't think that you will bulk up like men do if you practice these techniques. If you want a perfect slim zero flat belly follow the exercises and the diets that I am going to suggest to you in few moments. You will become and look slimmer if you do so.

Your clothes will fit better. And you will feel more confident when you're wearing your clothes or relaxing on the beach.

Both men and women can get six pack abs or flat belly. So how can you get a flat zero fat belly?

First you will have to exercise and eat the right foods. You can read my **free three cheat sheets** on the back pages of this book to find out more about the best foods that can help you to build your perfect belly. There are ways to build up your stomach muscles. And I am going to show you what you have to do.

But here is a word of warning. The exercises I am going to show you in a few moments are not a magic pill that can get you a zero fat belly overnight.

There are no short-cuts to gain the flat fat-free belly of your dream in a week. You have to be committed and be prepared to work hard to achieve this goal. The reality of getting the perfect flat belly involves hard work and dedication. And that's why you cannot lose weight by exercising or dieting alone.

If you are willing to work hard to have the body of your dream, then you will be able to achieve it.

Do you know why you want a perfect slim flat belly? Majority of people want the perfect abs for cosmetic purposes. They want to look their best when dressed or they want to show off their bodies while on the beach.

Some women celebrities pride themselves for having a perfect slim flat abdomen. They include stars of the motion picture industry and sports.

They pride themselves when they achieve their goals getting the perfect stomach because they know the hard work it takes to get defined zero fat-free muscles.

Generally women often prefer having less defined stomach muscles. By nature they have less fat than men.

Perfect belly is not only something to be proud of cosmetically. New medical studies also indicate that those who carry excess weight around their middle area are more at a risk of having heart disease and stroke. This goes for both men and women.

It is therefore desirable for both sexes to have flat abdomens and to carry less weight around their middle sections.

But if you think that you can get the perfect slim stomach through only sit ups and a crash diet, think again.

Getting the perfect slim belly requires training - real training which requires time and dedication to sculpt your abdominal muscles to the way that you want them to become.
If you are motivated then eventually you could achieve a perfect slim abs. If you are someone who easily gives up at the first sign of adversity, then you will have a difficult time achieving your goal. If you are prepared for hard work then you can achieve your perfect slim abs.
Before we move on to discuss next why you need to be having the right diet while building up your stomach muscles, let's recap on what you've read so far.

Summary of Chapter One:

1. Having a perfect six pack abs is when your abdominal muscles are so defined that they can be clearly seen.

2. While men prefer to have bulky six pack abs, women may choose to have flat fat-free belly. All meaning the same thing.

3. Some of the advantages of having a flat slim zero fat belly is while you're clothes fit better, you'll also feel more confident wearing them.

4. There are three free cheat sheets for you to read on the last page of this book. As you read these cheat sheets you will find out more about what you can eat including the best foods that can help you to build your perfect flat belly.

5. There are no shortcuts to gain fat-free slim belly. It requires commitment, a bit of hard work and dedication.

6. Having less fat around the middle area of the body reduces the risk of having heart attack and stroke.

7. Now let's discuss why you need to be on the right diet when striving to build your stomach muscles to be free from fat.

Chapter 2:

If You Read Nothing Else ... Read Chapter Two!

You have to watch your diet if you really want to have a perfect zero fat flat belly. And this is how you do it. Increase your intake of protein. And cut out on the carbohydrates. This does not mean you're going to lose a lot of weight. Rather you want to lose your belly fat.

If you are overweight, then reading this guide is an opportunity for you. Use these tips to reduce your weight and work towards sculpting your body. Not only will you look better, you will also feel healthier if you do so.

Foods that are high in protein are good for bulking up muscles. They are also good for losing fat. These types of foods tend to trick the body into thinking that it is getting more fuel while in reality it is actually receiving less. You should go on a high protein diet if you want to build and strengthen your abdominal muscles.

That's why body builders and athletes drink raw eggs. The reason for that is because there is lot of protein in raw eggs. They enhance the strength and stamina of athletes and body builders. And here are some foods which are high in protein:

1. Meats
2. Fish
3. Poultry
4. Nuts
5. Legumes
6. Eggs

Not only will these foods help you to get energy, they will also help you to bulk up your muscles. Foods that are fortified with protein are equally good. They include foods that do not normally contain protein but have protein added to them.

One of the best foods to eat when building muscles and is good for creating six pack slim abs is fish. You need to eat a fatty fish which is high in Omega 3 oils.

Fish is not only an excellent source of protein it is also good for the heart and the digestive tract. Eating fatty fish will also help to keep your brain healthy.

When you eat meat, skip sauces and bread. Just eat protein when you are on a high protein diet. Eating protein will give your body energy. It will also enhance your metabolism to burn fats. You will lose weight in your belly that way. By losing weight in your stomach area you will be able to build defined abdominal muscles.

Though eggs are also a good form of protein, you have to watch how you cook them. Hard boiled eggs are low in calorie and high in protein. That is a good way to start when you are trying to attain a perfect six pack slim fat-free stomach.

You can eat meat. But if you are not keen on meat, then eat legumes. Nuts are also a good form of protein. It is advisable that you eat a high protein-diet in the morning so that you can get your metabolism working.

Stay Away from These Foods

If you are determined to build a fat free slim belly then it is advisable that you stay away from certain types of foods. These types of foods include simple and complex carbohydrates.

Dairy is a product that is high in fat and you should eliminate it from your diet. You can include fibers by taking capsules. Bread and vegetables tend to be high in sugars. Exclude sugars from your diet when you are building a flat belly.

It is also important to eat all the foods on the food pyramid. It is never a good idea to eliminate one type of food over another for a long period of time. When you are building the perfect abs, you should concentrate on a high protein diet, but still eat vegetables as well as whole grains and dairy.

Sweets have no place in your diet as they do not offer any nutritional value whatsoever. Simple carbohydrates are absorbed quickly and do not stick around long enough to give your body any sort of nutrition.

Eliminate simple carbohydrates and starches from your diet if you want to have lean, rock hard perfect stomach.

Visit the link here below to watch Video One.

http://tiny.cc/ao7t7x

What Can You Drink?

You also need to watch what you drink when you are striving to build perfect belly. Drink water when you are building your perfect stomach.

Stay away from energy drinks. They are full of caffeine. Also avoid so-called health drinks as they are made from sugar and alcohol. Majority of drinks including alcohol contain sugar.

If you drink coffee or tea, then you shouldn't add sugar or cream. If you cannot tolerate the drink in that manner, then skip it altogether and have water instead.

Apart from its hydrating properties, water will also boost your energy levels.

How You Should Eat

You may remember I mentioned earlier that it is important that you eat more proteins if you want to achieve a perfect size of slim fat free abdomen. How you eat is very important and should not be taken lightly.

You should eat foods with high calorie content in the morning. The reason why you should do so is because your body will burn off the calories during the day while you are active.

You should not eat late at night. If you eat your meals late, the food will not be digested well. The food will stay longer in you as you are not physically active at night.

You should chew your food very well before swallowing it. When you chew your food properly you will find that you'll eat less and have fewer digestive problems.

Drink a glass of water before each meal. This will curb your appetite so that you eat less.

Once you are eating and drinking well, you'll be able to build your abdominal muscles which others will admire. Not only will you feel well within yourself, you'll also look healthy.

Visit this link below to watch Video 2:

http://tiny.cc/yt7t7x

Summary of Chapter Two

1. Increase your protein intake and cut down on eating carbohydrates if you want to lose weight.

2. Foods that are high in protein are good for building muscles.

3. Egg is high in protein and that's why body builders and athletes drink it raw.

4. Another best food for building muscles is fish.

5. In order to build a zero fat slim belly, do not eat certain foods such as dairy.

6. Stay away from energy drinks.

Chapter 3:

How to Train and Build Abdominal Muscles within 7 Days

You will have to exercise if you want to tone your abdominal muscles. There is no other alternative way to tone your abdominal muscles.

If you do not need to lose weight, you can still use the toning exercises as outlined here in this guide.

By toning your muscles, you will be able to sculpt your abdominal muscles in the way that you want.

If you are overweight and want to lose weight to get the sculpted muscles you wanted, then you still need to do toning exercises.

In addition you also need to do some cardiovascular exercises. I will show you later how to do these exercises.

Let's discuss toning first. Crunches are the ideal way to tone your abs. They are one of the many toning exercises that you should use on a daily basis to strengthened the muscles in your abdomen.

Crunches are the first exercise you want to incorporate into your daily routine so that you can have sexy stomach.

If you are a woman and want a flat abdomen but not the defined muscles like men it is possible. Women can get sexy, washboard abs without looking like a man.

Your abdominal area will be flat, but softer. Though the muscles will be defined, they will not be bulging like those you see in men. Both women and men get different results from exercise routines.

Using the tips and exercises you are reading now you can get your perfect abdomen whether you are a man or a woman.

Let's start. I am going to show you how to do abdominal crunches. Let's see how you can do centre crunches.

1. Lay flat on your back and bring your knees up so that your feet are flat on the floor.

2. Put your hands behind your head.

3. Raise your head and body. Then pull up your head and body towards your knees, concentrating fully on your abdominal muscles.

4. Gently lower your head and body back to its original position as you were before raising the head.

5. You should isolate the muscles as you are pulling up so that you feel the strain.

6. Repeat these crunches 8 times. On the first day, you may be able to do only two or three repetitions. Or you may only be able to do one.

If it has been a while since you have worked out, it will be more difficult for you to use these muscles. If possible try and repeat the crunches as many times as you can without hurting yourself. Stop the exercise if you are in a lot of pain.

You have to do the crunches in order to build your abdominal muscle. You build the muscle by tearing it a bit, and then let it heal. Then tear it again. That's why it is painful when you are doing crunches.

As you continue to do this exercise every day, you will notice that it becomes easier to do. And it will start to feel different. You will no longer feel the strain as long as you continue with the exercises.

The more you practice your crunches, the better toned your belly will become.

Now visit the link below to watch a session on how to do abdominal crutches.

http://tiny.cc/ex7t7x

While the crunches will flatten and tone your abdominal muscles, it is not the only the exercise (center crunches) that you need to do in order to get the perfect abs.

You also need to do side to side crunches.

How to do side to side crunches

Side to side crunches is to help you to develop the abdominal muscles on the sides of your abdomen. Just as you move up straight while doing the center crunches earlier, you move side to side when you do side crunches.

1. Lie flat on your back on the floor.

2. Start with one side. You can choose the left or the right hand side of your abdomen.

3. Pull yourself up to lean towards that side and return to the position where you started from.

4. Repeat this exercise 8 times, just as you did with the center crunches.

5. After you finished, repeat the exercise on the other side.

While doing the center and the side crunches, you must also do the following:

1. Allow your muscles to relax after each time you do your reps of crunches.

2. You want to take a few deep breaths and relax the muscles after you finish the toning.

3. When you are performing the crunches, however, you want to tense up the muscles, effectively isolating them so that they will get toned.

4. Another way to perform crunches for perfect abs is to lean on one side and then lift your body up, concentrating on the abdominal muscles. This technique will tone the muscles on the sides.

Remember that you want to work the entire abdominal area to achieve the look of a sculpted zero fat flat belly. You need to do both front crunches as well as side crunches as you lay on your back as well as your side to achieve this look.

Visit the address below to watch training Video 4.

http://tiny.cc/j47t7x

Crunches may seem difficult at first, but will soon become easier. You may want to increase your repetitions as you continue to work on your stomach so that they will continue to be effective.

The best aspect about using this type of toning exercise is that you will start to see the results of your efforts not long after you have started working on your abdominal muscles. You can usually see a difference in your muscle tone after a week of performing these exercises.

Try to do these exercises every day. If you skip a day, for some reason, just pick up where you left off the next day. Do not get discouraged if you get out of the habit. It is more important to get back into the habit as soon as possible.

Summary of Chapter Three:

1. If you want to tone up your abdominal muscles, then you will have to exercise.

2. If you are overweight and want to lose weight to get your flat slim belly, you need to start with toning exercises.

3. Doing crunches is the ideal way to tone your abdomen.

4. You will learn how to do center and side abdominal crunches.

5. Side to side crunches helps to develop the abdominal muscles on the sides.

Chapter 4:

How a Simple Leg Exercise Can Flatten Your Abdominal Muscles In 28 Days Or Less

You've just learned how to do crunches that can tone your abdominal muscles.

But crunches are not the only exercise that you need to do when you are looking for the perfect flat, fat-free belly.

In addition to doing crunches, you also need to use leg lifts to tone your abdominal muscles. You can do leg lifts at the same time as you do your crunches. Here's how to do your leg lifts.

a. Lay flat on your back on the floor.

b. Put your hands to your side with your palms down facing the floor.

c. Lift both legs up as high as you can, even if it is less than an inch off of the ground. While you are doing this, you need to once again isolate the muscles in your abdomen and tighten them up.

It is always good to work in repetitions of 8 when you are performing toning exercises.

The leg lifts will work well to tighten the muscles in your abdomen, making them looking defined.

Like you learned earlier about crunches, you will notice the results from this type of exercise within a week.

Visit this address below to view a video on how to do leg lift exercises.

http://tiny.cc/co8t7x

After you have done the two leg lifts, you can also do one leg lift at a time. This is often easier to do and will tighten your side abdominal muscles.

Do one leg at a time and then the other, repeating the exercise of each leg at a time. As you continue to do leg lifts for abs, you will notice that the leg lifts get easier.

You will be able to lift your legs higher and higher as you continue to practice the exercise.

When you get better at this type of exercise, you can also use weights on your ankles creating resistance when lifting your legs. You can purchase leg weights at a sports store.

Leg lifts and crunches are two of the toning exercises that you can use that will work towards tightening up your abdominal muscles. These exercises will work well in your effort to get the perfect flat stomach, but you must be able to do the exercises every day. It is important to concentrate on the muscles that you are toning while you are performing the exercises. By isolating the muscles and giving them total concentration, while working on this activity, you will find that the exercises not only get easier, but they start to produce results right away.

Next we are going to look at levitating lifts. But before you turn to the next chapter, here is the summary of this chapter.

Summary of Chapter 4:

1. While doing crunches, you also need to do a leg lift to tone up your abdominal muscles.

2. Leg lift exercises tighten the muscles in your abdomen making them looking defined.

3. Leg lifts and crunches are two of the toning exercises that you can use towards tightening up your abdominal muscles.

Chapter 5:

Learn the Secret to Build Zero Fat Belly Even If You're Overweight

Another toning exercise that you can use to flatten your belly as well as define the muscles is the levitating lift.

a.   Like the exercises described earlier, you need to lay flat on your back on the floor with your hands at your sides, palms facing down.

b.   You have to lift both your legs and your head up a few inches, while concentrating on your abdominal muscles.

This exercise is similar to the leg lifts. The first time that you attempt this exercise, you will most likely not be able to get much of your legs and head off the ground.   It will appear difficult and almost impossible at first, but as you continue working at it a number of times, you will eventually be able to lift up your head and your legs at the same time.

When you're doing this exercise, you will be exercising another part of the abdominal muscles and will further work towards sculpting them.

You use an exercise mat when doing this exercise. This is not only more sanitary to use, but is also more comfortable for your head and neck.

You should also do this toning exercises in repetitions of 8 each and work as many times as you can at a time. Even if you find it difficult, do not get discouraged.
If you are overweight, you need to lose weight before you can even see your abdominal muscles. You should concentrate first on doing the toning exercises.
They will help tone your muscles and can make it easier for you to lose weight. Toning exercises work well in combination with lower body cardiovascular exercises to give you best results.

Visit the address below to watch Training Video 6.

http://tiny.cc/7s8t7x

Summary of Chapter Five

1. Levitating Lift exercise is another exercise to use to flatten your abdominal muscles.

2. When you are doing Levitating Lift exercise, you are also exercising another part of your abdomen.

3. If you're overweight, you need to do toning exercises first to tone your muscles.

4. Toning exercises work effectively with lower body cardiovascular exercises.

Chapter 6:

Which of These 5 Cardio Training Workouts Would You Prefer?

In addition to the toning exercises that you have now learned, you also need to use cardiovascular exercises to work on the lower half of your body, which include your abdomen. There are many cardiovascular exercises that you can use for the lower half of your body.

If you are overweight and want to develop the perfect flat slim belly, then the first thing that you need to do is to start to lose some of that excess weight.

We have already talked about the need for eating proper diet and nutrition. Now we will discuss how to do cardiovascular exercises.

So what are these cardiovascular exercises?

Cardio exercises, for short, are exercises that get your heart pumping and will help you to lose weight fast.

Cardio exercises should be performed in the morning or as early as possible at the beginning of your day. When you do those exercises you will speed up the metabolic rate of your body. And as a result you will burn more calories during the day. These are some of the things you mustn't do.

 a. You should never perform cardiovascular exercises right before you retire to bed as you will find it difficult to go to sleep.

 b. You should never perform cardiovascular exercises after you have eaten or it can give you a stomach cramp.

If you cannot get up early in the morning to do your cardio exercises, then you should do them when you get home from work and before you eat.

This will help you to burn off calories and will also tone your lower body.

This is not to say that the cardio exercises that you do cannot work for your upper body, too. Some cardio machines will work on both the lower and upper parts of the body.
Others will tone the lower half of the body. You must make sure that whatever type of machine you use you will also tone the lower half of your body.

You can buy your own cardio machine or you can join a gym. You will find that gyms may offer many exercise machines that can help you to get the abs that you want as well as help you lose weight.

Even if you are not overweight, you should still exercise using cardiovascular machines for your abs. This will give you an intense workout that will help sculpt your abs faster and easier.

Some gyms charge a low monthly fee for membership. So effectively you will you have access to cardio machines that will help you to burn calories as well as tone up your lower body. I will discuss some of these machines in few moments.

But before that here are some of the cardio exercise machines that you can use which will tone up your lower half and as well as give you the abs that you want:

- Stair stepping machine

- Elliptical machine

- Rowing Machine

- Treadmill

- Exercise Bike

All those five cardiovascular machines will not only get you slimmer, they will also tone up your abdominal muscles.
Most people find a machine that they like and settle into a routine with it.

Stair Stepping Machine

The stair stepping machine was the exercise machine of choice in the 1980s and works very well as a cardiovascular machine as well as a lower body toner. You can get your abdominal muscles toned easily when you are using the stair stepper.

When you first start working on the stair stepper, you will find that it is difficult to stay on this machine for long. There are several types of machines.

Some of them actually have a rolling set of stairs that you have to climb while others simulate the climbing motion. Most stair stepping machines today are designed to display by showing you how many stairs you have climbed as well as how many calories you have lost.

The first time you are on a stair stepping machine you will find it hard to stay on it for more than five minutes, especially if it has been a while since you exercised.

If you feel lightheaded or dizzy when you are using the stair stepping machine, or feel short of breath, you need to stop the exercise immediately. Stair stepping is a high impact cardiovascular exercise. You should always discuss any new exercise routine with your physician before you start doing that exercise.

After you have used the stair stepper more often, you will notice that you can stay on it for longer periods of time. You do not need more than 20 minutes on the stair stepper each day to get the results that you want.

You can adjust the tension of the stair stepper to make it more difficult to use by increasing its resistance to suit your needs.

As you get better and better on the stair stepper, you can also attach leg weights to your ankles so that you can increase the tension as you climb. You can continue with this exercise routine as you work to sculpt your abs.

Concentrate on your abdominal muscles when you use the stairs. Your abs should be first and foremost your focus when you are using the machine.

Pull your abs in as you are using the stair stepper and keep them taut to gain maximum benefit.

In addition to exercising your abs, you will also notice that you'll get firmer legs, buttocks and thighs when you use the stair stepper in this way.

If you like the stair stepper, you may decide to buy one of these machines to use at home. You will find that the more you use the stair stepper, the better toned you will be and the more calories you will burn. It will also get easier to stay on the stair stepper for the full 20 minutes the longer you continue to use it.

Elliptical Machine

The elliptical machine will not only get your abs in shape, but will also exercise the lower half of your body as well as your upper half. The elliptical machine performs the motions of cross country skiing. This is a machine that is low impact and is easy to use.

It will allow you to move both your legs and your arms at the same time. It is one of the most effective ways to lose weight using a cardiovascular exercise machine. It can do you wonders when it comes to toning your abs.

The elliptical machine will be easier to use than the stair stepper as it does have a high impact. But equally it does the job.

You will start to notice the results right away. You will not feel too much out of breath compared to using the stair stepper.

Many people like using the elliptical machine because they can do so without the pain that other machines cause to their knees and back. The elliptical machine also allows you to move your arms back and forth, promoting more calorie burning energy. When you are using the elliptical machine, suck in your gut and tighten your abdominal muscles. You will feel the machine start to work on all of the muscles in your body.

When you concentrate on a certain set of muscles and tighten them as you are working out, you can expect to get better results in that area. The elliptical machine is a fun machine to use and will work well to tone almost every part of your body including the rock hard abs that you want.

Rowing Machine

The rowing machine is one way that you can also use to get your abdominal muscles to tighten up. It will also tone up on your legs, buttocks and arms. This is a high impact machine and will require you to mimic the motions of rowing a boat.

Rowing is an excellent way to lose weight. It will help you to burn calories. Someone who is in a reasonably good health and not severely overweight will enjoy the benefits of this machine.

Some of the modern rowing machines are equipped to display how far you have rowed and also allow you to race against other rowers.

Some of these machines can even show you how many calories you have lost and your heart rate when using this type of cardiovascular exercise machine.

The only disadvantage of using a rowing machine is that it could be hard on the knees. And that's why it is best for someone who is not obese and with no problem with their knees.

Here are some tips for you while you row. Suck in your abdominal muscles. And hold them in as you pull backwards and slowly relax the muscles as the machine pulls your body forward. By doing those things you will feel the tension pulling on your abdominal muscles. And as you continue to row, you will soon find that it gets easier and easier each time that you use the machine.

While you may find it difficult to continue rowing for a long time when you first start out, after you get the hang of this machine, you will find that it is easy to use and even entertaining. You may decide to get one for your home to keep your abs as well as your other muscles in shape.

Treadmill

The treadmill is one of the most popular of all cardiovascular exercise machines. It is used for walking as well as jogging and running. Anyone can use a treadmill. One of the best aspects about using the treadmill is that it can be used by anyone to tone up as well as to lose weight.

You should start out by walking on the treadmill and sucking in your abdominal muscles as you walk. Whenever you are exercising on the treadmill, you should concentrate on the muscles that you want to exercise and tone.

The treadmill will tell you how far you have walked as well as how many calories you have burned. It will also tell you your heart rate. Treadmill can be used for running, although it is just as effective at toning up your abdominal muscles when you walk.

The treadmills that you get today are much more advanced than those that were made many years ago. You may find that you like the treadmill so much that you decide to buy one for your home.

Exercise Bike

The exercise bike is also one way that you can tighten up your abdominal muscles. You will also lose weight while toning the lower half of your body.

You can get an exercise bike which allow you to sit straight up and down, or one in which you recline and have your legs in the air.

Both of these exercise bikes are useful for toning up your abdominal muscles.

The new exercise bikes that are on the market, as well as in the gym, are able to tell you how far you have ridden and how many calories you have burned.

The new exercise bikes will allow you to race against other riders that are shown on the LCD screen. This can give you an added incentive if you need some motivation to keep pushing on when you are exercising. This can make using this piece of cardiovascular exercise equipment easy and fun.

Whenever you are using cardiovascular exercise machines, you should make sure that you are in good health before attempting the routine. You should talk it over with your doctor and see if you are healthy enough for an exercise routine.

If you feel any pain, dizziness or light-headedness, you should stop exercising. This is something that can be a danger signal.

Start out your cardiovascular exercising slowly so that you can gradually work your way up. Try and work to the point to keep your body trim and healthy. Using an exercise bike can also tone up your abdominal muscles.

Summary of Chapter 6:

1. Cardio exercises are those exercises that get your heart pumping and will help you to lose weight fast.

2. Cardio exercises should be performed in the morning as early as possible at the beginning of your day.

You should never perform cardiovascular exercises right before you retire to bed, as you will find it difficult to sleep.

3. Cardiovascular exercise machines will not only get you slimmer, they will also tone up your abdominal muscles.

Chapter 7

The Secret of Building a Flat Zero Fat Belly Is Simply Knowing and Using Proven Workout Exercise Routines

You will notice, when you go to your gym, that there are weight machines that are made to exercise the abdominal muscles.

Like the other machines you learned about earlier, weight machines will keep your abdominal muscles in shape as well as tone and define them.

When you are using the weight machines for your abs, you should use them every other day.

You do not want to bulk up your abdominal muscles. What you want is to tighten up your muscles so that they look toned and defined.

There are several weight machines at the gym that you can use to strengthen your abs and tone up your muscles so that you can have a perfect zero fat belly.

Machines that work well will cause you to twist and tighten your abdominal muscles and enable you to mimic the sit up routine.

Because you can adjust the weights and tension on these machines, you can expect good results if you use them every other day to tone up your muscles.

Before you use any type of weight machine at the gym, you need to know how to use them. Most gyms will have instructors to teach you how to use the machines.

The instructors will show you the right way to use the exercise machine safely in order to get the best results. Using a weight machine incorrectly can cause injuries.

Talk to your gym instructor before you start using the machine. Ask them how you can use the machine so that it tightens up your abdominal muscles. The instructor may even have other machines that you can equally use for the same purpose. When you first start using the weight machines, you will want to use the lowest tension level or weight. Do repetitions of the motion as instructed and try to do 3 repetitions of 8.

Sometimes you may not think that the weight machine is doing you any good, but chances are that you will feel tension in your abdominal muscles the day after you exercise.

You can wait for a day and then perform the same exercises again. The least of what you want is to strain your muscles when you are using the weight machines causing injuries to yourself. You should just aim to create a little tension as possible in your abdominal muscles.

After a week of using the weight machines with success, you can then gradually increase the weights. With persistence and repeating the exercises, it will gradually become easier. Be sure to use both the twisting motion weight machines to exercise the side abdominal muscles as well as the front abdominal muscles when you are using the sit up machine.

Each week, increase the level of the weight, building tension on your abdominal muscles.

As you persist with the exercises, you will soon start to notice a change in the tone of your muscles. If you belong to a gym, you will want to try all of the weights that may be available.

If you have a home gym, be sure to use your weight machine the right way to prevent causing injury to your muscles.

Now you can visit the link below to watch the Training Video 7.

http://tiny.cc/yz8t7x

Summary of Chapter 7

1. Weight machines will keep your abdominal muscles in shape as well as tone up your abdominal muscles.

2. The trick about using weight machines is to use them every other day.

3. You do not want a bulky six pack abdominal muscles like men do – what you want is to tighten up your muscles so that they looked toned and defined.

4. Before using any weight machine, you must know how to use them to avoid injuries or damaging your abdominal muscles.

5. Make sure to use both the twisting motion weight machines to exercise your side abdominal muscles as well as the front abdominal muscles when you are using a sit up machine.

Chapter 8:

How This 75 Year Old Dance Routine Can Sculpture and Flatten Your Belly to Lose Fat

Pilates are a type of toning exercise that has been used by dancers for nearly 75 years.

One way that you get involved in Pilates is to join a class. This is another way that your local gym can help you.

Pilates are excellent when it comes to toning up muscle, especially the abdomen. If your gym offers a Pilates class, try and sign up.

Pilates work well when it comes to teaching you how to isolate certain muscles and how to get them toned. Not only will your Pilates class work on the abdomen, it will also have impact on other muscles as well.

Once you get the hang of the Pilates and how to use them, you can use this exercise routine to work on your abdomen when you are at home.

There are many people who are glad to teach Pilates to others so they can learn this type of toning exercise.

Pilates will let you concentrate on your muscles which you want to tone and exercise them to the maximum.

Throughout this guide, I kept explaining the importance of isolating muscles and concentrating on them when exercising. This apply to all machines – be it a cardiovascular machine, a toning exercise machine or a weight machine.

You're probably wondering how you can learn to do this. Pilates can teach you how to focus on your muscles and make the most of your workout.

Pilates are much more concentrated type of exercise than any other toning exercise routine. There are number of reasons why many people like to use Pilates to sculpt their abdominal muscles. Here are some of these reasons.

One of such reasons is because you can get the same results from a 15 minute workout as you can get from a 45 minute traditional workout. Pilates are made to concentrate on muscles and tone them so that they are strong as well as sculpted.
If you are at a loss as to how you can learn Pilates' exercises or do not know a gym where you learn it you may learn it from watching a DVD, which you can rent from your local video store.
Once you learn Pilates, chances are that you will use them in other exercise routines.

Pilates are low impact exercises and less likely to tone up your abs as compared to the impact it would have on the rest of your body. If you want to have the best looking abdomen, try Pilates. Many fashion models and others who exhibit perfect abs swear by this exercise routine. You will notice a big change in your body when you begin practicing Pilates. You will not only exhibit a perfect abdomen, but you'll have perfect toned muscles in other parts of your body.

If you want to achieve the perfect abdomens, you owe it to yourself to try Pilates - one of the best forms of exercise for toning muscles. That brings us to the next training video. Visit the link here to watch Training Video 8.

http://tiny.cc/x18t7x

Summary of Chapter 8:

1. Pilates are a type of muscle toning exercises.

2. Pilates are excellent when it comes to toning up muscles especially in the abdomen.

3. Once you know how to use Pilates properly, you use this exercise routine anywhere even while you are at home.

4. Pilates will let you concentrate on the muscles which you want to tone and you will be able to exercise them to the maximum.

5. Pilates have many advantages, for example you will be able to get the same results from a 15 minute workout as you will get from a 45 minutes traditional workout.

6. Pilates will not only tone your abdominal muscles, you will also have a perfect toned muscle in other parts of your body.

Chapter 9:

Do You Easily Give Up Your Dream – Having A Zero Fat Belly?

As you are working on your abdominal muscles, you will sometimes feel you've reached a stalemate. You may feel your abdominal muscles are not getting any more defined.

It's the same feeling experienced sometimes by people who diet. Everyone who is trying to lose weight or trying to tone their muscles will reach a point where they'll feel that they cannot get any further with their efforts.

They may feel disappointed because of the fact that they are doing everything possible but do not seem to achieve the results they wanted.

So what do you do when you feel you reach a plateau and cannot lose any more weight or gain any improvement in your muscles?

The best way that you can avoid this problem is to change the way you are doing things. Sometimes, your body gets used to a certain routine to the point where you cannot get it to perform any more.

When this happens, the only thing you can do is to change your workout routine. If you have been using only Pilates instead of machine weights, it's advisable to start using them too. Start changing the toning exercises as well and begin using another cardiovascular machine. This jolt may be just what your body needs in order to get back into shape. You need to make some changes.

You should also watch your diet at this time. You may want to start eating smaller meals more often in an effort to get more energy into your body. This is one change that you can make that will help you attain your goals.

Summary of Chapter Nine:

1. How to manage your disappointment anytime you feel you have reached a stalemate. You may be feeling you cannot lose any more weight or gain improvement in your muscles.

2. Overcome your disappointment by changing your workout exercise routines.

3. Watch your diet at this critical time. Start eating smaller meals more often in an effort to get more energy into your body.

Chapter 10:

Using Supplements? The Sooner You Know The Better

Enhancement supplements are used by body builders, including those who want to have perfectly well formed abs, as a way to bulk up muscle growth.

Natural enhancement supplements work by increasing the blood flow into the muscles. It allows you to get more from your workout. You can often get a more intense workout when you use enhancement supplements than if you just workout without them.

Natural enhancement supplements are made with herbal ingredients that have been used for hundreds of years as a way to increase energy levels in the body. Anyone who is looking for a way to increase blood flow to muscles can use these natural enhancement supplements. You should not confuse natural enhancement supplements with steroids. Steroids are products that are created from synthetic hormones and should only be taken under the supervision of a doctor.

Many people who work out and want to build muscle bulk enjoy using enhancement supplements as part of their workout routine. Natural enhancement supplements can make it easier to work out harder for a longer period of time.

They also give you better results from your workout routine.

Other people dislike the idea of using enhancement supplements because they do not produce the instant bulk or muscle growth that they expect. Many people who feel this way do so because they have confused natural enhancement supplements for working out with steroids.

Steroids are usually illegally obtained. They should be avoided by anyone who wants to stay healthy. The side effects of taking steroids include increased aggression, organ damage and even mental instability.

Men will notice their testicles shrinking from taking steroids and women will begin to grow hair on their faces and chests. Steroids are an unnatural enhancement that many in the body building circuit use to get those large, unnatural looking muscles.

Six pack abs or zero fat slim bellies are not unnatural looking. They are a well-defined muscle group in your abdominal region. You do not have to resort to any artificial means to achieve the perfect six pack or fat free belly. You can get these abs using the exercises and diet formulas demonstrated in this guide without having to resort to any artificial supplements.

If you want to accelerate your workout then take natural supplements that contain herbal ingredients. This will not do you any harm and may also give you a psychological boost as well.

You can purchase natural enhancement supplements at health food stores as well as at some online outlets. Remember to ONLY take natural supplements and stay away from steroids.

There is no magic pill that you can take to get the perfect abs or a zero fat belly. You can only acquire a perfect six pack abs or a zero fat belly through hard work and dedication.

If you are willing to dedicate time to exercise and eat a proper diet you will definitely get a perfect six pack abs or a zero fat flat belly.

But if you are looking for a way to get this look without any type of effort on your part, think again. No enhancement or magic pill is going to do it for you. Hard work and discipline will allow you to have the perfect abdomen of your dream.

Summary of Chapter 10:

1. Learn the difference between natural and artificial enhancement supplements.

2. Natural enhancement supplements are made of herbal ingredients, probably have been used for hundreds of years as mean of increasing energy levels in the body.

3. Natural enhancements supplements are not the same as artificial supplements like synthetic hormones such as steroids.

4. Steroids are artificial enhancement supplements and may cause serious side-effects such as increased aggression, organ damage and even mental instability. Stay clear of artificial enhancement supplements.

5. To achieve a perfect zero fat flat belly, hard work, dedication and discipline cannot be replaced by use of artificial supplements.

Chapter 11:

How to Keep Your Stomach Muscles Fat Free Even If You Feel Like Giving

It stands to reason that once you have achieved the perfect abs or fat free belly you will want to keep it.

Once you get to the point where you are happy with the way that your abdominal muscles look, you want them to stay that way.

You should continue to eat the right way, lead a healthy lifestyle and workout regularly. This is a good lifestyle choice for anyone - regardless of whether or not they have the perfect abs or a fat free flat belly.

Many people who achieve this type of feat feel that they cannot ever stray from their routine without their perfect abs collapsing and turning to fat. While you will want to stay on your routine as much as possible and eat healthy foods, if you stray from your diet or fail to show up for the gym, do not panic. This does not mean that you will lose the perfect abs that you worked so hard to attain. Keeping the perfect abs is more of a mind-set than anything else. You will want to continue to diet and exercise and be mindful of the way that you look. Chances are that if you achieved the perfect abs of your dreams, you have already demonstrated a remarkable amount of determination and ability to achieve a goal.

You might even feel a little bit let down, now that the goal has been completed. Or you might think that you do not have to do anything to maintain this new body.

You should never feel let down because you have completed a goal. While the initial quest to achieve the goal can be very inspiring for many people, and get them all revved up to complete the goal, you can still have other goals that you can set your mind on that can give you a feeling of achievement.

You should still keep to your exercise routine as you are working out so that you can continue to keep the firm abs.

If you feel that you can let your body go and you abandon your exercise routine because you have achieved your dream, think again. You could have a difficult time getting back into shape if you let your perfect abs go to waste. Or shall we say waist? This is because your abdominal muscles will turn to fat if not used.

It is important that you continue exercising and maintaining your perfect abs that you have worked so hard to achieve.

It is not a good idea to fight hard to get the perfect abs for the summer so that you can look good in a bathing suit and then let yourself go during the cold months so that you can eat whatever you want and not exercise. This is not only for your body, but it will make things even more difficult for you when next summer when you want once again to attain the perfect abs.

While there is nothing wrong to indulge now and again, you do not want to break your routine to the point where you have to start all over again from scratch in achieving the perfect abs when you want to get in shape in the near future.

Once you have achieved the perfect abs, you will feel good about yourself and will also want to stay that way.

One way that you can do this is to take a picture of yourself with your perfect abs. Post the picture on the refrigerator so that you are constantly reminded of how hard you worked to achieve it.

Visit here to watch Training Video 9.

http://tiny.cc/048t7x

Summary of Chapter 11

1. Once you achieve your perfect six pack or zero fat flat belly, you should continue to eat the right way, lead a healthy lifestyle and workout regularly.

2. If you do stray away from your routines – your diet, exercise or fail to show up for your gym – do not panic. Try and get back to your exercise routines.

3. Keeping the perfect abs is more of a mindset than anything else. You will want to continue to diet and be mindful of the way that you look.

4. You might feel a little bit let down that you have achieved your goal or you may be thinking that you do not have anything to maintain your new body.

5. As a cardinal rule, you should never feel let down because you have completed a goal.

6. You should still keep up your exercise and other routines so that you can continue to keep your firm abs muscles intact.

Chapter 12

Would You Pass This Psychological Test?

Achieving the perfect abs or a fat free firm belly can do more for you mentally and psychologically than any other part of your body.

Sure enough, your body will be looking good. You will also look healthy. You will feel good about your health and happy about the way that you look in your clothes.

But the way that you feel mentally will be even better than the way that you feel physically. This is because you will have a renewed sense of self confidence. Not only because you are happy with the way that you look, but because you have set a goal for yourself and achieved that goal.

Few things enhance the confidence level more than setting a goal and completing a goal. This will make you feel like a worthwhile person and give you a higher sense of self- esteem.

If you want to feel good about yourself, one way to do so is to set a goal and follow through with that goal. The psychological impact of attaining the perfect abs will be enormous.

There is also a psychological component to achieving the perfect abs or a slim flat belly that you need to explore when you are trying to achieve this goal. How bad do you want it? You need to ask yourself how bad you want to have the perfect abs and what you are willing to go through to get them.

In order to achieve this goal, you need to want it very badly. Many people will complain that they cannot lose weight or cannot quit smoking or find a new job or a new partner. They are usually defeating themselves when they say these things.

Instead of telling yourself that you want to lose 20 pounds, tell yourself that this is your ultimate goal, but your goal for the next week is to lose 2 pounds. Begin your regimen of diet and exercise and you will easily lose the 2 pounds.

You will feel good about yourself as you have achieved a small goal on the way towards a larger one.

The same way of thinking must be used when you are trying to achieve the perfect six pack abs or a zero fat abs. When you have reached the goal of your ideal weight and you are ready to define your abs so that you have the perfect six pack or slim flat abs, start to break the goal down into smaller goals.

It is often too overwhelming for someone to only focus on the large goal when they are trying to attain a big improvement in their life. And a perfectly sculpted body is a big improvement. Instead of looking at the entire picture, break it down. Set your smaller goals so that you can achieve the large one by saying that your goal for this week is to make it to the gym every day and achieve a certain number of reps or maintain a certain amount of time on a machine.

One of the best aspects about the cardiovascular exercise machines is that they can give you results right away as to how much time you have spent on them, the calories you have burned and the workout you achieved.

If you try to attain a little bit more each time, you will not only be working towards your goals, but you will also feel good about yourself.

You will find that by exercising regularly and eating healthy foods you will start to develop a positive mindset as it is. Exercise is like a wonder drug and can rejuvenate you. You will notice that you have more energy and feel better about yourself when you are exercising your way towards the perfect six pack abs. Your entire body will feel and look healthier.

It may take a couple of months before you can achieve the six pack abs or zero fat abs that you want, depending on your current weight and health. But if you set small goals for yourself and work towards achieving those goals, you will continue to feel motivated about having the perfect six pack or slim flat abs.

Occasionally, you might indulge in something that is not good for you or skip an exercise. If this happens, do not let it deter you from your goal. One of the reasons why many people fail to achieve their goals is because they give up the first time they encounter adversity.

They go off the wagon by eating something that they should not eat or not exercising for a day or two and figure out that they should just give up. People who diet or try to quit smoking also make this mistake. One of the biggest secrets to having the perfect abs is that you cannot give up. If you fall off the wagon, just jump back on it again. Do not beat yourself up over a failure because that is self-defeating.

Hang a picture of the perfect six pack abs or flat belly where you can see it every day so that you can continue to work towards your goal. Motivate yourself with small rewards for a job well done. Do that by giving yourself small gifts or treating yourself to something that you like each time you reach a goal.

Once you have taken the steps outlined in this guide to achieve the perfect abs or belly, you can use the same type of goal oriented motivation to achieve other areas of greatness in your life. As you achieved a goal, you can use the same strategies to achieve other goals too.

Anything is possible if you have dreams, ambition and goals. If you are willing to do what it takes to move towards that big goal by accepting the challenges of smaller goals and overcoming them, then you have what it takes to do just about anything that you set your mind to in life. Including getting the perfectly sculptured body and gorgeous six pack abs or fat free belly!

Summary of Chapter 12:

1. The way you feel mentally will even be better than the way you feel physically once you achieved your goal of the perfect abs or having slim flat a belly.

2. If you want to feel good about yourself – one way of doing that is to set a goal and take steps to achieve it.

3. Before you set a goal for anything, first ask yourself how badly do you want to achieve that goal. Think about what you have to go through to achieve it.

4. To achieve any goal – whether big or small, you need to want it very badly. It is only by feeling that way that you will be driven to achieve it. To successfully achieve any ultimate goal you set for yourself, the   secret to reach that goal is to break into smaller goals.

5. Hang a picture of the perfect six pack or flat belly where you can see it every day so that you can continue to work towards your goal.

6. Anything is possible if you have ambitions, dreams and goals.

7. If you are willing to do what it takes to move towards that big goal by accepting the challenges of smaller goals and overcoming them, then you have what it takes to do just about anything that you set your mind on to achieve in life.

BONUS PAGES
CHEAT SHEET ONE

How You Can Achieve Ten Healthy Eating Habits

Dear Reader

First, thank you for deciding to buy my book, 'Building Your Lean Zero Fat Belly – Simple Abs Muscle Workout Training Exercise Routines for Women'.

I want to help you achieve your goals much faster by reading and applying what is in these three cheat sheets in addition to what you probably have already read in the book. So this is one of the three cheat sheets I have specially written for you.

As you know already, a habit can be either good or bad. And it can certainly become a way of life. So which habits? It's about how you eat. It's up to us as individuals to choose whether or not we want healthy eating habits and make them part of our daily lives.

When we view healthy eating habits as a choice and not something that has been forced upon us, we have the power to incorporate those healthy eating habits into our way of life. With power and freedom to choose, healthy eating habits can simply be our everyday eating habits and not something we will ever have to think about again.

So how can we do that? Well here some steps we can take:

Add something new to your diet. Strangely, we tend to associate diet with taking something out of our diet. It doesn't have to be that way. If you try and add something new to your diet every day, you will not feel as though you are missing anything. Try a new fruit or vegetable that you have never tried before.

Eat a good breakfast that has high fiber content. A simple act as including whole grains will keep you full and fit for the entire day. If you are concerned about cholesterol, an egg white frittata can fit the bill.

Have a snack. For some unknown reason we tend to decrease our intake of calories and forget that the point of staying healthy is not to starve ourselves but to nourish ourselves. Snacking in-between meals (healthy snacking of course) is the way to keep your metabolism up and running.

Increase your fluid Intake – For some women, water does not go down very well. Try different variations of liquid beverages until you find the one that is right for you. Sometimes simply adding fruits such as orange, lemon, or lime to your water will give you the added flavor you desire. Even green tea with honey added to it can make the difference.

Mix it up a little bit. Have fun. If you get bored with salad, feel free and be creative. Creating a different salad for every day of the week is easy when you mix it up a little bit. Adding things like hard-boiled eggs, broiled chicken, garbanzo beans and anything else you can think of can give the standard salad a pick-me-up. Cranberries and oranges are wonderful additions to a tossed salad.

Watch the clock – Become a time management expert when it comes to healthy eating habits. Once you have finished dinner, have whatever snack or cup of tea that you desire shortly thereafter. There is nothing wrong treating yourself to hot cup of cocoa once in a while. Just make sure you don't stuff your stomach full too close to bedtime.

A little organization goes a long way. By preparing a few simple items on a Sunday afternoon, you can make your healthy eating habits a breeze. An egg white vegetable quiche can be sliced into smaller portions and eaten for breakfast on the go during the week.

Broiling a chicken breast and adding tomato, lettuce, and fat-free mayo can be lunch two to three times per week. This will help you resist the urge to buy something "quick" on the run. It is healthy and you prepared it. You save time, money, and you are eating healthily at the same time.

Are you someone who deprives yourself? Everyone craves a treat once in a while. Do not deprive yourself. Just be picky about what you choose. Denying yourself will only make you eat the whole pie instead of just a piece. Dark chocolate is a healthy treat that offers mood boosters and important vitamins and minerals. It does not hurt that it tastes great too. So why not have a go at times?

Don't forget to exercise. Just like eating healthily, include exercise into your life just as you do with your eating habits. While exercise is not a healthy eating habit, one without the other will not work. Exercise does not have to be something you dive into at full speed. Starting off slowly, perhaps power walking with a friend, is all the momentum you will need to get and keep this healthy habit in place.

Grab a partner – Sometimes when we set off to do something

alone, we find it hard to keep motivated. Incorporating a healthy eating habit partner into your plan will allow you to have someone you have to be accountable to as well.

Try these 10 healthy eating habits, make them your daily routine, you will be surprised how fast these habits become your second nature.

CHEAT SHEET TWO

5 Natural Foods You Can Include In Your Weight Loss Plan

Have you ever tried to lose weight? Did you realize there so many over-the-counter supplements, diet pills, and weight loss remedies? Yes they are and from my own experience it is easy to get confused and overwhelmed.

And the most worrying part is that most of those weight-loss remedies are full of chemicals which can be harmful to your immune system. Though they may offer you a quick fix on how to lose weight, chances are that the weight will come back on just as quickly as it came.

But it doesn't have to be that way. You'll be amazed that without taking weight loss supplements, natural foods can help reduce your weight, maintain it and help keep to it off. By turning to natural foods, not only do you lose the weight, you also increase your metabolism and boost your health. Now that you aware of these benefits, why not we explore these five natural foods that you can add to your diet to promote and keep off that weight?

1. Salad – While not everyone loves the greens, when you look at the multitude of benefits a green, leafy salad has to offer, you might just change your tune. Salads, especially those with green leafy spinach, can provide antioxidants such as vitamins A, E, and C while giving you extra folate as well. The beauty in a salad, however, comes in the creation. A salad can be anything you want it to be. You can add sunflower seeds, chicken, or even fruit like tangerines.

2. Good old-fashioned chicken soup – For many years, studies have shown that chicken soup has all the ingredients to boost your immune system, shorten the duration of a cold, and help promote weight loss. The reasoning behind the weight loss seems to be the fact that soup simply fills you up. And, when you fill up your soup with beans for fiber and chicken for protein along with vegetables for antioxidants, you are naturally and effortlessly achieving many weight-loss goals. If your stomach is feeling full, you are less likely to binge.

3. Lean beef and chicken – Beef that is lean can promote weight loss as it provides the right amount of protein that a dieter needs. Also, amino acids found in extra lean beef can assist with losing weight and maintaining muscle mass. Chicken, with the skin removed, is low in fat, high in protein and tastes great too. Meat and chicken can always be added to a salad for an all-around weight-loss benefit.

4. Oats and whole grains – The fiber in oats and whole grains offers a full and satisfying feeling, which in turn allows you the opportunity to eat less. Rolled oats and those that have the least processing done to them are the most beneficial as they are all-natural and fill you up quickly and healthily.

5. Beans – Eating beans such as kidney, lentil, and cannellini offer the benefits of fiber and protein all rolled into one.

Beans can be eaten in a fajita mixed with lean beef or chicken, or made into healthy casserole or even tossed into a salad. Not only are these foods ideal for losing weight, they are tasty and versatile as well. Try them and you'll never look back.

CHEAT SHEET THREE

Discover 5 Healthy Foods That Can Change Your Day

Isn't it rather strange that majority of us doesn't view food as our source of power? Our attention and focus tends to be rather on the fear of every possible ailment we could think of. Worries about aches, pain, mood and many others. We do not look up to food as our source of power?

Nature provided us with everything including food to maintain our health throughout our lifetime.
Every food has its benefits. And here are five foods that are worth mentioning:

1. Chicken – It's made of white meat which contains the essential vitamins B12, B6, and B3. Chicken lowers our risk of stroke. It boosts our moods. Chicken is low in fat (especially with the skin removed) and high in protein. Besides its nutritional benefits, chicken is versatile. It can be cooked in so many ways using a variety of tools such as the outdoor grill or an indoor rotisserie. And the B vitamin it provides has many benefits such as:

1. Fighting off anemia
2. Maintaining healthy blood cells
3. Preventing heart disease
4. Increasing energy
5. Boosting the immune system
6. Converting carbohydrates into energy

2. Broccoli and salads – Broccoli and salads, especially salads made with leaf spinach, have many benefits. Broccoli contains vitamins A, C, and E while spinach provides folate, which helps to maintain and produce newer healthier cells for the body. Vitamins such as A, C, and E help to boost the immune system; this could mean less time off sick and shorter duration of ailments such as the common cold.

3. Bananas – Offers as sweet treat any time during the day. You can reach for a banana whenever you wish. Bananas have numerous uses. You can choose to eat a banana as it is, or you can add it to a yogurt or a bowl of multi-grain cereal. Either way, you will gain the benefit of a quick energy booster that can sustain you for several hours alongside with the mood-altering benefit of the B6 vitamin.

4. Dark chocolate – The good news is that good quality, dark chocolate has many benefits to help make you feel great. The cocoa in chocolate has heart-healthy benefits such as lowering your cholesterol and reducing heart disease. That is not all; dark chocolate can lift your mood significantly with its tryptophan and magnesium. Grabbing a piece of high quality dark chocolate will not only help your heart, it will also help your mind.

5. Whole grains – Whole grains have been found to contain selenium which has been shown to significantly reduce depression. Whole grain breads with your favorite spread or even an all-natural peanut butter provide fiber, selenium, and protein. The nice thing about whole grains is that you can mix and match whole grain breads with different spreads and come out with a variety of healthy foods that make you feel great in the end.

QUESTIONS OR COMMENTS?

Thank you for having faith in me and decided to buy my book. I hope you find the contents helpful and informative. I'd love to hear your thoughts. Email me at danny.agbet@gmail.com

One Last Thing ...

When you turn to the next page, Amazon will give you the chance to rate this book and share your thoughts through an automatic feed to your Facebook and Twitter accounts. If you believe you have gain something valuable out of this book, I will feel very privileged if you could spare few minutes of your time and post your thoughts – share with your friends.

If you feel particularly strong about the contribution this book made to your life, I would be eternally grateful if you post a review on my book page on Amazon.

Thank you and all the best,

Daniel

End

DISCLAIMER AND/OR LEGAL NOTICES: Every effort has been made to accurately represent this book and it's potential. Results vary with every individual, and your results may or may not be different from those depicted. No promises, guarantees or warranties, whether stated or implied, have been made that you will produce any specific result from this book. Your efforts are individual and unique, and may vary from those shown. Your success depends on your efforts, background and motivation.

The material in this publication is provided for educational and informational purposes only and is not intended as medical advice. The information contained in this book should not be used to diagnose or treat any illness, metabolic disorder, and disease or health problem. Always consult your physician or health care provider before beginning any nutrition or exercise program. Use of the programs, advice, and information contained in this book is at the sole choice and risk of the reader.